YOUR KNOWLEDGE HAS VALUE

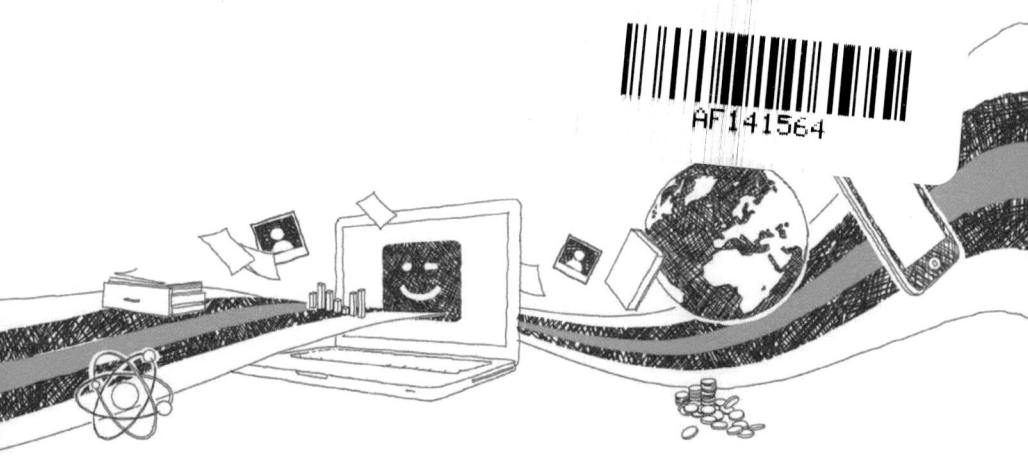

- We will publish your bachelor's and master's thesis, essays and papers

- Your own eBook and book - sold worldwide in all relevant shops

- Earn money with each sale

Upload your text at www.GRIN.com and publish for free

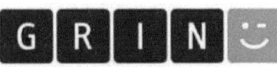

Ajit Kulkarni, Manish Bhatia

Design of Regioselective Bilayer Floating Tablets of Propranolol Hydrochloride and Lovastatin for Biphasic Release Profile

GRIN Publishing

Bibliographic information published by the German National Library:

The German National Library lists this publication in the National Bibliography; detailed bibliographic data are available on the Internet at http://dnb.dnb.de .

Imprint:

Copyright © 2014 GRIN Verlag GmbH
Print and binding: Books on Demand GmbH, Norderstedt Germany
ISBN: 978-3-656-85555-2

This book at GRIN:

http://www.grin.com/en/e-book/284893/design-of-regioselective-bilayer-floating-tablets-of-propranolol-hydrochloride

GRIN - Your knowledge has value

Since its foundation in 1998, GRIN has specialized in publishing academic texts by students, college teachers and other academics as e-book and printed book. The website www.grin.com is an ideal platform for presenting term papers, final papers, scientific essays, dissertations and specialist books.

Visit us on the internet:

http://www.grin.com/

http://www.facebook.com/grincom

http://www.twitter.com/grin_com

Design of Regioselective Bilayer Floating Tablets of Propranolol Hydrochloride and Lovastatin for Biphasic Release Profile.

Ajit S. Kulkarni*, Manish S. Bhatia[1]

* Satara College of Pharmacy,
  Plot no. 1539, Additional MIDC, Degaon,
  Satara, M.S., India PIN- 415004.
[1] Bharati Vidyapeeth College of Pharmacy,
  Kolhapur, M.S., India

ABSTRACT

The purpose of the study was to design bilayer floating tablets of Propranolol hydrochloride and Lovastatin to give immediate release of Lovastatin and controlled release of Propranolol hydrochloride. Bilayer floating tablets comprised of two layers, immediate release layer and controlled release layer. Direct compression method was employed for formulation of the bilayer tablets. Short term accelerated stability studies were carried out on the prepared tablets. All the formulations floated for more than 12h. More than 90% Lovastatin was released within 30 min. from the formulations. HPMC K4M and Xanthan gum retarded the release of Propranolol hydrochloride from the controlled release layer for 12h. After stability studies, apparent degradation of both the drugs were found but the drug content was found to be within the range. Diffusion exponent (n) was determined for all the formulations (0.53-7). Based on coefficient of correlation(R), the release of Propranolol hydrochloride was found to follow mixed release pattern of Hixson-Crowell, Korsmeyer-Peppas and matrix, except formulation F6 and F9, which followed zero order release pattern. Statistical analysis revealed that there was no significant difference in in vitro release pattern of the drugs before and after stability studies.

Key words: Lovastatin, Propranolol hydrochloride, floating, bi- layer tablets.

INTRODUCTION

Hypertension and hypercholesterolemia frequently coexist and may require concomitant drug treatment. The efficacy and safety profile of Lovastatin given in the presence of antihypertensive medication was evaluated using patient subgroups identified in the Expanded Clinical Evaluation of Lovastatin study.[1-3] The treatment of hypertension co-existing with hyperlipidemia is always subjected to various kinds of drugs, like, angiotensine converting enzyme inhibitors, calcium channel blockers, β-blockers etc. Control over the blood pressure was effectively achieved in combination therapy than individual therapy. In U.S., ever large clinical trials were conducted namely Antihypertensive and Lipid Lowering Treatment to Prevent Heart Attack Trials (ALLHAT). Several studies suggest that hypertension & hyperlipidemia may have additive or perhaps synergistic effects. Various clinical trials conducted suggest combination therapy for the treatment of hypertension & hyperlipidemia.[4-7] In the present study, we have attempted to combine Lovastatin and Propranolol hydrochloride by formulating into a bilayer tablet. Many approaches are currently utilized to design gastroretentive dosage forms[8,9].These include, low density floating dosage forms [10] ; high density dosage forms which remain at the bottom of the stomach, bioadhesive systems[11]; swelling sytems [12]; hydrodynamically balanced systems[13].Gastric retention of the drugs provide advantages such as (i) delivery of the drugs with narrow absorption windows in the small intestinal region; (ii) longer residence time in the stomach could be advantageous for local action in the upper part of small intestine[13]. Various dosage forms have been designed for gastric retention; these include, floating tablets [14]; floating beads [15]; pellets [16]; floating granules [17]; floating microspheres [18]. The current investigation employs development of floating bilayer tablet for different release pattern of Lovastatin and Propranolol hydrochloride using gas generating agent. Propranolol hydrochloride, a non-selective beta adrenergic blocking agent has been widely used in the treatment of angina pectoris, hypertension and many other cardiovascular disorders. The drug is water soluble and has half life of 3.4 h. It's bioavailability is 5-50% [19].Therefore, it was chosen as a drug for preparation of gastro-retentive formulation. Lovastatin, a HMG Co-A reductase inhibitor is widely used in the treatment of hyperlipidemia. The drug has very short half life of 1.1-1.7h with very less bioavailability 5-50% [20, 21]. The bilayer tablet comprised of immediate release layer of Lovastatin and controlled release layer of Propranolol hydrochloride. The release kinetics of Propranolol hydrochloride was analyzed using different mathematical models. Accelerated stability

3

studies were carried out on the prepared tablets [22]. At the end of stability studies, tablets were evaluated for in vitro drug release, floating characteristics, drug content and other physicochemical parameters.

MATERIALS AND METHODS

Propranolol hydrochloride was procured from CIPLA Ltd., (Mumbai, India).Lovastatin was a generous gift from Panacea Biotech (Chandigarh, India). HPMC K4M and Xanthan gum(XG) were obtained as gift samples from Panacea Biotech (Chandigarh, India).Sodium starch glycolate(SSG), was procured from Okasa Pharma Ltd., (Satara, India).Tablettose 80 was received as a gift sample from Wockhardt Ltd.,(Aurangabad, India).Other materials were purchased from commercial sources:Magnesium stearate(Loba chemicals, Mumbai, India), di-calcium phosphate(S.D.Fine chemicals,Mumbai,India), Sodium bi carbonate(Research lab, Mumbai, India).

Method

Preparation of Bilayer Floating Tablets

Bilayer floating tablets were prepared by direct compression method employing sodium starch glycolate as superdisintegrant, HPMC K4M and XG as rate controlling polymers, sodium bicarbonate as gas generating agent. The optimum concentrations of above ingredients were developed under experimental conditions and on the basis of trial preparation of the tablets. Preparation of bilayer floating tablets had two steps: i) preparation of controlled release layer

The ingredients (Table 1) were accurately weighed and were added into the blender in ascending order. The powder mix was blended for 20 min. so as to have uniform distribution of drug in the formulation. 300 mg of the powder mix was weighed accurately and fed into the die of single punch machinery (Cadmach, Ahemedabad, India.) and compressed at 1.5 N compression force using 10 mm concave punches. ii) preparation of immediate release layer

The ingredients (Table 1) were accurately weighed and were added into the blender in ascending order. The powder mix was blended for 20 min. so as to have uniform distribution of drug in the formulation. 100 mg of the powder mix was weighed accurately and fed onto the controlled release layer and compressed at 3 N compression pressure using 10 mm concave punches.

4

Floating characteristics

Floating characteristics of the prepared formulation were determined by using USP 23 paddle apparatus [19] (Electrolab TDT-06P, Mumbai, India) at paddle speed of 50 rpm in 900 ml 0.1N HCl (pH 1.2) at 37 ± 0.2^0C for 24 h. The time between introduction of tablet and its buoyancy on the simulated gastric fluid (floating lag time) and the time during which the dosage form remain buoyant (floating duration) were measured. Also, the integrity of the tablet during study was observed visually (matrix integrity).

Drug content

Propranolol HCl

Twenty tablets were accurately weighed and average weight was calculated. These tablets were ground to a fine powder. An accurately weighed tablet powder equivalent to 120 mg of Propranolol hydrochloride was dissolved in methanol and volume was made to 100 ml. The solution was filtered through Whatmann filter paper No.41. An aliquot of 1 ml was taken and diluted to 24 ml. Further, 1 ml from this diluted stock solution was taken and diluted to 10 ml. For the estimation of Propranolol hydrochloride from the sample solution absorbance of sample solution was recorded at 255nm and 287nm and the quantity of Propranolol hydrochloride in the sample solution was obtained from the calibration curve. The calibration curve for Propranolol hydrochloride was plotted using absorbance of 10 standard solution of Propranolol hydrochloride over a concentration range of 1mcg/ml to 10mcg/ml. Lovastatin has no absorbance at 255nm and 287nm.

Lovastatin

Twenty tablets were accurately weighed and average weight was calculated. These tablets were ground to a fine powder. An accurately weighed tablet powder equivalent to 50 mg of Lovastatin was dissolved in methanol and volume was made to 100 ml. The solution was filtered through Whatmann filter paper No.41. An aliquot of 1 ml was taken and diluted to 100 ml. For the estimation of Lovastatin from the sample solution a difference spectrophotometric method was developed and validated to eliminate interference of absorbance by Propranolol hydrochloride in the sample solution. The calibration curve for estimation of Lovastatin was obtained by plotting difference of absorbance at 247nm and 312nm of 10 mixed standard solution containing 1mcg/ml to 10 mcg/ml of Lovastatin against its concentration.

Drug release

The release of Propranolol hydrochloride and Lovastatin from different formulations was determined using USP 23 paddle apparatus2 [23] (Electrolab TDT-06P, Mumbai, India) under sink conditions. The dissolution medium was 900 ml 0.1N HCl (pH 1.2) at 37 ± 0.2^0C with a stirring speed of 50 rpm. For each formulation, the study was carried out in triplicate. The release data was analyzed to study release kinetics using zero order, Korsmeyer-Peppas and Higuchi equations [24, 25].

Hardness

Hardness of the prepared formulations was determined using Monsanto hardness tester (n=10) [26].

Stability

To assess the drugs and formulations, short term stability studies were carried out. All the formulation samples, sealed in aluminium packaging coated inside with polyethylene, and various replicates were kept in humidity chamber maintained at 40^0C and 75% RH for 3 months. At the end of the studies, samples were analyzed for drug content, floating characteristics, hardness and in vitro dissolution studies. The study was carried out in triplicate.

DSC studies

Thermal analysis was carried out using Mettler Toledo 821^e DSC (Switzerland). The tablet was ground to powder and 1-2 mg sample was hermetically sealed in an aluminum pan and heated at a constant rate of 10^0C/min, over a temperature range of 50^0C-500^0C. Inert atmosphere was maintained by purging nitrogen gas at the flow rate of 20mL/min.

Assessment of Similarity factor

The similarity factor (f2 factor) was used to compare dissolution profiles of Propranolol hydrochloride. The in vitro dissolution release profile of the formulations before stability studies were considered as reference and in vitro dissolution release profile of the formulations after stability studies were considered as test. Similarity factor was calculated using PCP Disso software. The f2 factor is a logarithmic reciprocal square root transformation of the sum of squared error. The f2 factor is used to quantitate agreement between two dissolution profiles. Dissolution testing was conducted under exactly the same

6

conditions. The values of *f2* in between 50 to 100 shows similarity in dissolution profile with reference.

$$f_2 = 50 \times \log \left\{ \left[1 + (1/n) \sum_{j=1}^{n} |R_j - T_j|^2 \right]^{-0.5} \times 100 \right\}$$

Statistical Analysis

Analysis of variance (ANOVA) was performed to find out significant difference in drug released at 12h, floating lag time and drug content from all formulations. Student's 't' test was applied to assess difference in the release pattern of the drug before and after stability studies.

RESULTS

Floating characteristics

All the formulations floated more than 12h with lag time of 16 min. During floating duration formulations maintained matrix integrity (Table 2). Swelling of the tablets was observed, which added the floating ability to the formulations. A 5% concentration of sodium bi carbonate was found to be optimum for low lag time and prolonged floating duration. Floating duration and lag time was found to be the functions of amount of polymers incorporated in the formulations

Drug content

Propranolol hydrochloride (99.36%-102%) and Lovastatin (95.9%-102.02%) content were found within the specifications. Additives in the formulations did not have any effect on the drug content (Table 2).

In vitro drug release

Lovastatin

Immediate release layer of bilayer floating tablet disintegrated liberating Lovastatin. All the formulations liberated more than 90% Lovastatin within 30 min. A 8% concentration of sodium starch glycolate was found to be optimum. Disintegration of the immediate release layer did not have any effect on the characteristics of the controlled release layer.

Propranolol hydrochloride

Formulations liberated Propranolol hydrochloride more than 80% at 12h period (Table 3). The effect of Xanthan gum at different concentrations ranging from 20%-40% on the release of Propranolol hydrochloride from tablet matrices was observed. Figure 1 shows the release profile of drug from Xanthan gum matrix. Figure 2 shows release profile of drug from HPMC K4M matrix at different concentrations of polymer. Figure 3 exhibits release profile of drug from combined Xanthan gum and HPMC K4M matrices. All aforementioned polymers at different concentrations alone and in combination, release more than 80% drug in 12h period, indicating that the polymers could retard the release of the drug from matrices. It was also observed that, Xanthan gum retarded the release of the drug than HPMC K4M. Diffusion exponent 'n' values (0.53-0.7) indicated that the release mechanism is non-fickian or anomalous transport. The release data was fitted to different kinetic models and based on coefficient of correlation (R) best fit model was determined. (Table 4). Formulation F6 and F9 followed zero order model while other formulations followed either Korsmeyer-Peppas or Higuchi model or Hixson-Crowell model.

Hardness

Hardness (Table 2)for all formulations was found between 4-4.5 kg/cm^2. Hardness upto 4.5 kg/cm^2 was found to be optimum and did not affect floating characteristics and drug release.

DSC studies

DSC curves showed that there was no any incompatibility between Propranolol hydrochloride and Lovastatin. A peak was obtained at 171.39^0C for Lovastatin and at 164.27^0C for Propranolol hydrochloride (Fig.7). Combined DSC of Lovastatin and Propranolol hydrochloride shows peak at 168.82^0C. There is a small variation between the combined peak of Lovastatin and Propranolol hydrochloride and peaks of individual drugs. This variation can be due to close melting points of these two drugs or experimental error.

Stability studies

Floating characteristics

Tablets subjected for stability studies showed increased lag time upto 6 min. All the formulations floated for more than 24 h and showed good matrix integrity (Table 4).

Drug content

Propranolol hydrochloride (95.5%-100.91%) and Lovastatin (94.24%-101.41%) content of all the formulations was found to be decreased than original formulation. This may be because of apparent drug degradation during stability studies (Table 2).

Drug release

Lovastatin

There was no significant effect on immediate release of Lovastatin from immediate release layer. Drug release was found to be above 90% within 30 min. from all formulations(Table 3).

Propranolol hydrochloride

Decreased percent drug release was observed from all the formulations as compared to original in vitro drug release data. No significant difference was observed between the release pattern of bilayer tablets before and after stability studies.

Hardness

Hardness of the bilayer tablets was found to be increased to 4.4-4.7 kg/cm^2. This may be due to absorption of trace quantity of moisture during accelerated stability studies. This increased hardness did not have any significant effect on drug release.

Similarity factor

All the formulations showed similarity factor as shown in Table No.3. $f2$ value of Formulation F1 was found to be 90.12.

DISCUSSION

On contact with dissolution medium, hydrochloric acid in the test medium reacted with the sodium bi carbonate in the controlled release layer of the bilayer tablet, inducing CO_2 formation. The generated gas bubble was trapped in the matrix of the polymer and was well protected by gel formed by hydration of polymers. A 5% concentration of sodium bi carbonate was found to optimum to impart floating characteristics to the system. It was observed that concentration of sodium bi carbonate more than 5% led to fast reaction with formation of dispersion of the tablet. Hardness upto 4.5 kg/cm^2 was found optimum to impart compactness to the system. Gel formed by polymers alone and in combination was effective for the protection of gas bubble. Further, an increase in bulk volume, presence of internal voids in the dry center of tablet (porosity) made the tablet float on the test medium for 12-24h. During floating all the formulations showed good matrix integrity, which may be because of the compactness of the system, which is necessary to prevent the sweep of the table in lower part of gastrointestinal tract during interdigestive myloelectric cycle (Phase I-Phase II). As the concentration of the polymers was increased (F1-F9), it was observed that floating lag time was decreased and floating duration was increased. This can be explained as: As the concentration of polymers was increased there was more gel formation and easy trap of gas bubble in the matrix resulting in decreased lag time. As a function of time, a firm gel was formed increasing the volume of the tablet and decreasing density which resulted in more prolonged floating duration.

Uniform content of the drugs in the formulations indicates presence of labeled amount of drugs. Additives in the formulations did not have any effect on the active ingredients. Also, there was no any incompatibility between two drugs. This was further supported by DSC studies.

On immersion of bilayer tablet in the dissolution medium, immediate release layer disintegrated liberating Lovastatin with fine dispersion. Super disintegrant, sodium starch glycolate swelled by absorbing liquid medium leading to disintegration of the layer without affecting any characteristics of controlled release layer. 8% concentration of sodium starch glycolate was found to be optimum. 10% concentration of sodium starch glycolate disintegrated the immediate release layer but with the formation of flakes than fine dispersion, which is undesired for rapidly disintegrating tablets.

Formulations (F1, F2, F3) containing different concentration of Xanthan gum retarded the drug release as a function of concentration of polymer for 12h (fig.1). Xanthan gum, a hydrophilic polymer upon contact with aqueous fluid, is able to form quite viscous gel, and hence retard the drug release from hydrophilic matrix. Formulations (F4, F5, F6), containing HPMC K4M as polymer could retard the drug release for 12 h by the formation of viscous gel (fig.2). Xanthan gum showed higher ability to retard the drug release than HPMC K4M in identical formulations and experimental conditions. The release of the drug from xanthan gum matrices followed almost time independent kinetics while release from HPMC K4M matrices followed time dependent kinetics [27-29]. Under identical experimental conditions, the drug diffusivity in HPMC K4M gel higher than in xanthan gum gel. This difference in hindered transport of drug molecules within the two polymers brings out the real cause for the reported higher retarding ability of drug release from a xanthan gum matrix tablet than a HPMC K4M matrix tablets. Formulations (F7, F8, F9) containing combination of polymers did not give any synergistic effect of retarding drug release from the matrices when compared with drug release from individual polymer matrices. Formulation F7 released 97.1% drug at 12h period (fig.3). As concentration of Xanthan gum was increased (F8), keeping concentration of HPMC K4M constant, 8% drug retardation was achieved. Further, increase in Xanthan gum concentration did not increase much drug retardation from matrix. This indicates that, increase in polymer concentration increases drug retardation upto a certain concentration value after which, no increase in drug retardation is possible. [30]. With all formulations, a burst effect was observed that could be attributed to dissolution of water soluble Propranolol hydrochloride from the surface of the tablets [31,32]. Yet, this effect was least with HPMC-containing formulations. This finding could be explained by the hydrophilic nature of HPMC. When exposed to dissolution medium, the solvent penetrates into the free spaces between macromolecular chains of the polymer. After salvation of the polymer chain, the dimensions of the polymer molecule increase due to the polymer relaxation by stress of the penetrated solvent. This phenomenon is defined as swelling and is characterized by the formation of a gel-like network surrounding the tablet. This swelling and hydration property of HPMC causes an immediate formation of a surface barrier around the matrix tablet, which reduces the burst release [23]. Diffusion exponent 'n' value obtained (0.53-0.7) for all the formulations indicates that release mechanism was non fickian or anomalous transport of drug (coupled diffusion/ polymer relaxation) (24). This can be explained as: Propranolol hydrochloride is a hydrophilic drug in hydrophilic polymer matrix. The drug release from hydrophilic matrix is governed sequentially by the following processes: 1. hydration and swelling of the polymer which results in formation of gel; 2. dissolution of drug in hydrated matrix/gel; 3. diffuse out of the drug molecule through that hydrated matrix; and finally 4. surface erosion and/or dissolution of that formed gel –matrix. Diffusion of drug was the main mechanism of the release of drug from hydrated matrix.

After stability studies, lag time upto 14 min indicates the possibility of reaction of small concentration sodium bi carbonate with moisture during stability studies. But, there was no effect on the floating duration and matrix integrity of the tablets. Apparent drug degradation was found, but it was not significant. Decreased drug release was found from all the formulations. But, drug release complies the standard of release of drug as per the official standard, as more than 80% drug release was achieved. The statistical analysis of dissolution data before and after stability studies was carried out. Student's t-test was applied to assess the effectiveness of formulations. No significant change was observed in percent release data before and after stability studies for three months. Based on the release data, floating characteristics and similarity factor $f2$ value, formulation F3 was found to be an optimized formulation.

Analysis of variance showed significant difference in drug release at 12 h and floating lag time from all formulations F1-F9, at $P<0.05$ level. There was a non significant difference in drug content of the formulations F1-F9, at $P>0.05$ level.

CONCLUSION

Bilayer floating tablets for different release profile for different drugs can be formulated using HPMC K4M and Xanthan gum, alone and in combination to give controlled release of the Propranolol hydrochloride and sodium starch glycolate to give immediate release of Lovastatin. Hence, this dosage form should be further evaluated so that it would deliver two drugs from a single dosage form. This could improve patient compliance and give better disease management.

ACKNOWLEDGEMENT

Authors are thankful to Principal, Satara College of Pharmacy, Satara for providing laboratory facilities for carrying out this research work.

REFERENCES

[1] J.L.Pool, C.L.Shear, M.Downton, H. Schnaper, S. Stinnett, Lovastatin and coadministered antihypertensive/cardiovascular agents, Hypertension. 19 (1992) 242-248.

[2] R.Rubin, S. Silbiger, L. Sablay, J. Neugarten, Combined Antihypertensive and Lipid-Lowering Therapy in Experimental Glomerulonephritis, Hyper ahajournal. (2007) 92-95.

[3] A.Faggiotto, R. Paoletti, Statins and Blockers of the Renin-Angiotensin System, Hypertension. 34 (1999) 987-996.

[4] B.R. Davis, J.A. Cutler, D.J. Gordon, et al. Rationale and design for the antihypertensive and Lipid-lowering treatment to prevent Heart attack trials (ALLHAT), American J Hypertension, 9 (1996) 342-360.

[5] www. Lomasin .com

[6] S Oparil, Antihypertensive and Lipid-lowering treatment to prevent Heart attack trial, Hypertension, 41 (2003) 1006-1009.

[7] K.L Margolis, L.B. Piller, C.E. ford , Blood pressure control in Hispanics in Antihypertensive and   Lipid-lowering treatment to prevent Heart attack trial, Hypertension, 50 (2007) 854.

[8] S.Garg, S. Sharma, Gastroretentive Drug delivery Systems, Pharmatech. (2003)160-166.

[9] S.S.Davis, Formulation strategies for absorption windows, DDT, 10 (2005) 249-257.

[10] A. Streubel, J. Siepmann, R. Bodmeier, Floating microparticles based on low density foam powder, Int. J. Pharm. 241 (2002) 279-292.

[11] A.J. Moes, Gastroretentive dosage forms, Crit. Rev. Ther. Drug. Carrier. Sys. 10(1993) 143- 195.

[12] E.A.Klausner, E.Lavy, M.Friedman, A. Hoffman, Expandable gastroretentive dosage forms, J. Control. Release. 90 (2003)143-162.

[13] J. G. Rocca, H. Omidian, K. Shah, Progress in Gastroretentive Drug Delivery Systems, Pharmatech. (1998) 152-156.

[14] S.Baumgartner, J.Kristl, F.Vrecer, P.Vodopivec, B. Zorko, Optimisation of floating matrix tablets and evaluation of their gastric residence time, Int. J. Pharm., 195 (2000) 125-135.

[15] B.Y.Choi, H.J.Park, S.J.Hwang, J.B.Park, Preparation of alginate beads for floating drug delivery system: effects of CO2 gas- forming agents, Int. J. Pharm. 239 (2002) 81-91.

[16] S. Sungthongjeen, O. Paeratakul, S. Limmatvapirat, S. Puttipipatkhachorn, Preparation and in vivo evaluation of a multiple-unit floating drug delivery system based on gas formation technique, Int. J. Pharm. 324 (2006) 136-143.

[17] S. Shimpi, B. Chauhan, K.R. Mahadik, A. Paradkar, Preparation and   evaluation of Diltiazem hydrochloride-Gelucire 43/01 floating granules prepared by melt granulation, AAPS PharmSciTech. 5 (2004) 1-6.

[18] A. Srivastava, D.N. Ridhurkar, S.Wadhwa, Floating microspheres of cimetidine: Formulation, characterization and in vitro evaluation, Acta. Pharm. 55 (2005) 277-285.

[19] C.Dollery, Therapeutic Drugs, Churchill Livingstone, Edinburgh, 1999, pp. P259-P265.

[20] C.Dollery, Therapeutic Drugs, Churchill Livingstone, Edinburgh, 1999, pp. L105-L109.

[21] K.D. Tripathi, Essentials Of Medical Pharmacology, New Delhi, India, Jaypee Brothers Medical Publications, 2003, pp. 145.

[22] United States Pharmacopoeia 23, US Pharmacopoeial Convention, Rockville, (1993) 951.

[23] Stability testing guidelines. Stability testing of new drug substances and products, ICH guidelines.(2003)

[24] J.Siepmann, N.A. Peppas, Modeling of drug release from delivery systems based on hydroxypropyl methylcellulose (HPMC), Adv.Drug. Deli.Rev. 48 (2001) 139-157.

[25] P.Costa, J.M.S. Lobo, Modeling and comparison of dissolution profiles. Eur.J.Pharm.Sci. 13 (2001) 123-133.

[26] Banker, Theory and Practice of Industrial Pharmacy, Varghese Publishing House, Bombay, (2001) pp. 298-301.

[27] M.M. Talukdar, R. Kinget, Swelling and drug release behaviour of Xanthan gum matrix tablets, Int. J. Pharm. 120 (1995) 63-72.

[28] M. M. Talukdar, R. Kinget, Comparative study on Xanthan gum and hydroxypropylmethyl cellulose for controlled-release drug delivery.II. Drug diffusion in hydrated matrices, Int. J. Pharm. 151 91997) 99-107.

[29] S.Conti, L.Maggi, L.Segale, E.O.Machiste, U.Conte, P.Grenier, G.Vergnault, Matrices containing NaCMC and HPMC 2.Swelling and release mechanism study, Int. J. Pharm. 333 (2007) 143-151.

[30] H. Mehrgan, S.A. Mortazavi, The release behavior and kinetic evaluation of Diltiazem HCl from various hydrophilic and plastic based matrices, Iran. J. Pharm. Res. 3 (2005) 137-146.

[31] S.B. Tiwari, T.K. Murthy, M.R. Pai, P.R.Mehta, P.B. Chowdary, Controlled release formulation of tramadol hydrochloride using hydrophilic and hydrophobic matrix system, AAPS Pharm. Sci. Tech. 4 (2003) 31.

[32] M.S. Reza, M.A. Quadir, S.S. Haider, Comparative evaluation of plastic, hydrophobic and hydrophilic polymers as matrices for controlled-release drug delivery, J. Pharm. Pharmaceut. Sci. 6 (2003) 282-291.

Table 1. Formulation of bilayer tablets.

Immediate Release Layer

Ingredients	F1	F2	F3	F4	F5	F6	F7	F8	F9
Lovastatin	50	50	50	50	50	50	50	50	50
Tablettose80	41	41	41	41	41	41	41	41	41
SSG	08	08	08	08	08	08	08	08	08
Mag. stearate	1	1	1	1	1	1	1	1	1
Total	**100**	**100**	**100**	**100**	**100**	**100**	**100**	**100**	**100**

Controlled Release Layer

Ingredients	F1	F2	F3	F4	F5	F6	F7	F8	F9
Propranolol HCl	120	120	120	120	120	120	120	120	120
Xanthan gum	60	90	120	---	---	---	--	--	--
HPMC K4M	---	---	---	60	90	120	--	--	---
HPMC K4M	---	---	---	---	---	---	30	30	30
Xanthan gum	--	--	--	--	--	--	15	30	45
Mg.Stearate	2	2	2	2	2	2	2	2	2
Sod. bicarbonate	15	15	15	15	15	15	15	15	15
Dicalcium phosphate	15	15	15	15	15	15	15	15	15
Tablettose 80	88	58	28	88	58	28	103	88	73
Total	**300**	**300**	**300**	**300**	**300**	**300**	**300**	**300**	**300**

All fig. mg.
Total weight of the single bilayer tablet = 400mg.

Table 2. Evaluation of Physicochemical parameters.

Form. Code	Drug content %±s.d.				Hardness(kg/cm²) n=3		Floating characteristics					
	Prop. HCl n=3		Lovastatin n=3				Lag Time (min)		Floating Duration(h)		Matrix integrity	
	a.	b.	a.	b.	a.	b.	a.	b.	a.	b.	a.	b.
F1	100.92±3.5	95.5±2.3	102.02±6.8	101.13±8.3	4.1±0.15	4.4±0.11	8	10	13	13	+	+
F2	100.92±7.4	95.5±2.32	99.43±2.6	98.55±7.9	4±2.1	4.5±0.1	5	7	19	16	+	+
F3	99.37±1.3	97.82±2.32	96.85±2.6	95.96±3.9	4.3±0.15	4.6±0.15	2	3	24	24	+	+
F4	100.91±7.4	97.04±1.33	98.57±3.9	101.41±2.7	4.4±0.11	4.7±0.14	9	12	14	13	+	+
F5	100.14±4.6	96.27±3.54	96.85±2.5	100.26±7.5	4±0.15	4.4±0.11	6	8	18	15	+	+
F6	99.36±48	100.14±4.0	95.99±3.9	94.24±2.6	4.2±0.14	4.5±0.1	1	3	24	24	+	+
F7	102.46±6.1	96.27±1.33	98.57±4.8	95.13±1.48	4.5±0.15	4.6±0.12	10	14	14	13	+	+
F8	100.14±46	100.91±3.5	101.16±3.9	98.55±7.9	4.4±0.11	4.6±0.1	6	7	17	14	+	+
F9	99.36±4.8	97.82±2.32	100.3±5.6	97.69±8.3	4.1±0.12	4.5±0.05	2	4	24	24	+	+

a. Before stability studies
b. After stability studies
+. Very good

Table 3. In vitro release profile

Formulation Code	% Propranolol HCl released at 12 h %±S.D.	%± S. D[b].	% Lovastatin released at 30 min %±S.D.	%± S. D[b].	Similarity factor (f2)for Propranolol HCl
F1	100.43±0.64	99.5±3.2	101.33±7.08	99.78±7.08	90.12
F2	93.24±4.1	92.51±3	99.78±11.6	98.24±8.0	84.26
F3	87.53±2.3	85.68±3.5	102.87±4.63	101.33±10.7	89.61
F4	98.95±4	95.26±1.1	104.41±2.68	99.78±2.6	83.66
F5	91±3.2	88.08±3.8	99.78±7.08	95.15±2.6	86.10
F6	85.14±2.6	82.55±1.1	102.87±9.27	101.33±7	87.41
F7	99.87±1.9	96.36±0.55	102.85±4.63	101.33±5.3	79.39
F8	91.77±2.7	86.6±2.5	99.78±10.7	98.24±4.6	77.19
F9	85.14±2.6	81.82±4.9	101.33±5.35	96.69±2.6	76.42

b. After stability studies
n=3

Table 4. Model fitting for Propranolol hydrochloride.

Formulation Code	Matrix		Zero order		Korsmeyer-Peppas			Hixson-Crowell		Best fit
	R	k	R	k	R	k	n	R	k	
F1	0.9800	26.6	0.9466	9.15	0.9776	23.6	0.54	0.9821	-0.05	Matrix
F2	0.9817	24.8	0.9351	8.5	0.9822	22.6	0.54	0.9765	-0.04	Peppas
F3	0.9665	21.8	0.9590	7.6	0.9680	18.8	0.56	0.9722	-0.03	Hixson-Crowell
F4	0.9700	24.5	0.9489	9.9	0.9690	22.1	0.53	0.8569	-0.05	Matrix
F5	0.9720	22.9	0.9682	7.9	0.9821	18.36	0.6	0.9745	-0.03	Peppas
F6	0.9596	20.5	0.9802	7.1	0.9731	15.1	0.63	0.9783	-0.03	Zero order
F7	0.9791	25.5	0.9499	8.7	0.9810	22.8	0.54	0.9019	-0.05	Peppas
F8	0.9710	22.9	0.9734	7.9	0.9905	17.16	0.63	0.9737	-0.04	Peppas
F9	0.9569	20.4	0.9873	7.1	0.9849	13.27	0.7	0.9807	-0.03	Zero order

Fig.1

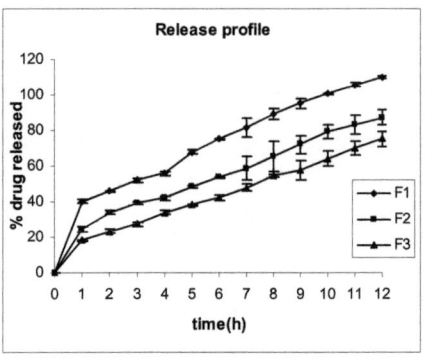

Fig.2

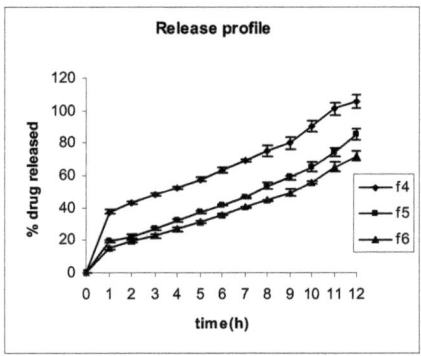

Fig.3

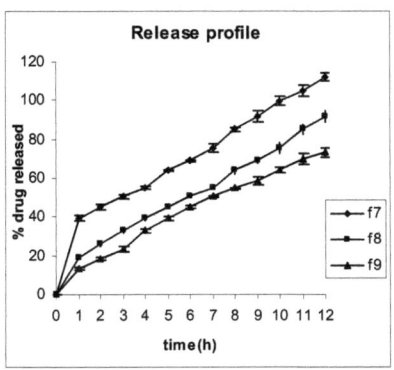

Fig.4

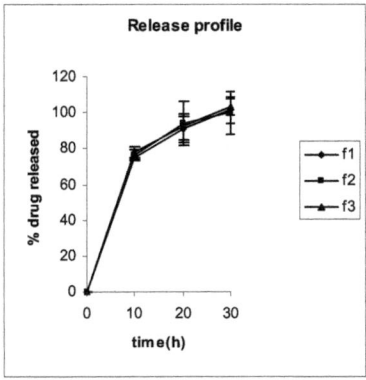

Fig.5

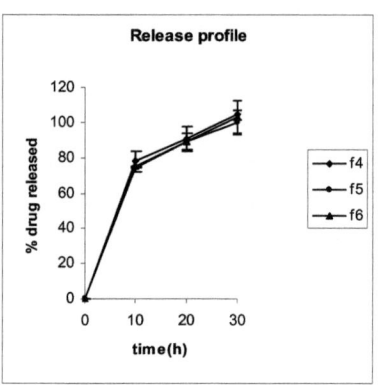

Fig.6

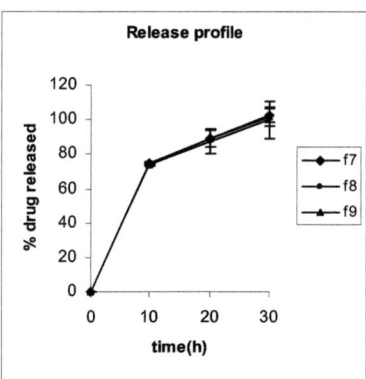

Fig. 7

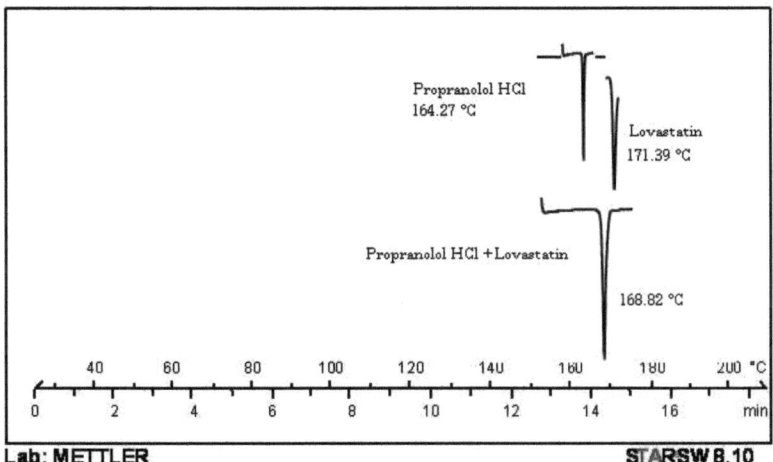

Propranolol HCl
164.27 °C

Lovastatin
171.39 °C

Propranolol HCl +Lovastatin

168.82 °C

40   60   80   100   120   14U   16U   18U   2U0 °C

0   2   4   6   8   10   12   14   16   min

Lab: METTLER   **STARSW 8.10**

FIGURE LEGENDS:

Figure 1. In vitro release profile of Propranolol hydrochloride from formulations (F1, F2 & F3 with Xanthan gum 20%, 30% & 40% respectively).

Figure 2. In vitro release profile of Propranolol hydrochloride from formulations (F4, F5 & F6 with HPMC K4M 20%, 30% & 40% respectively).

Figure 3. In vitro release profile of Propranolol hydrochloride from formulations (F7, F8 & F9 with Xanthan gum and HPMC K4M combination1:0.5, 1:1 & 1:1.5 respectively).

Figure 4. In vitro release profile of Lovastatin from formulations (F1, F2 & F3).

Figure 5. In vitro release profile of Lovastatin from formulations (F4, F5 & F6).

Figure 6. In vitro release profile of Lovastatin from formulations (F7, F8 & F9)

Figure 7. DSC combined thermogram of Propranolol HCl and Lovastatin